# Healthy and Happy Kids

## :: a wellness workbook for parents ::

I0435316

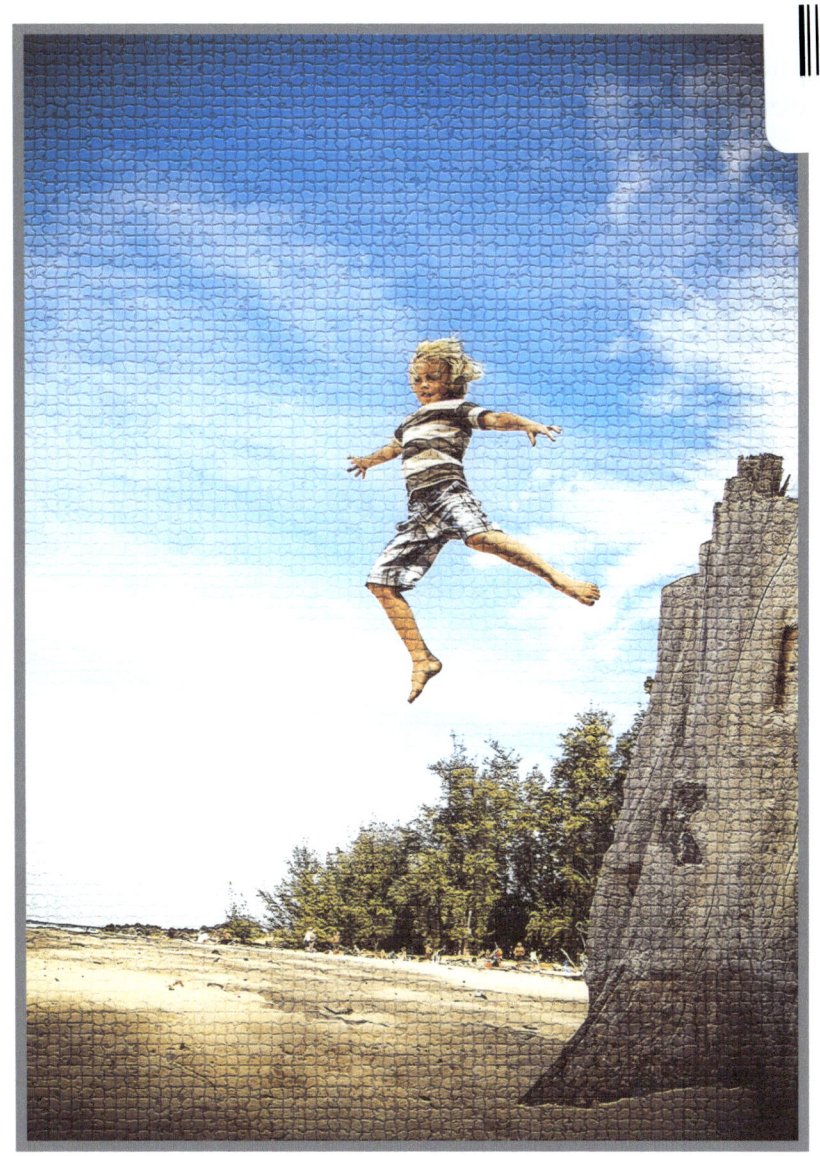

**by Kristin M. Mills, M.S., M.A.**
*Breathe & Be Wellness*

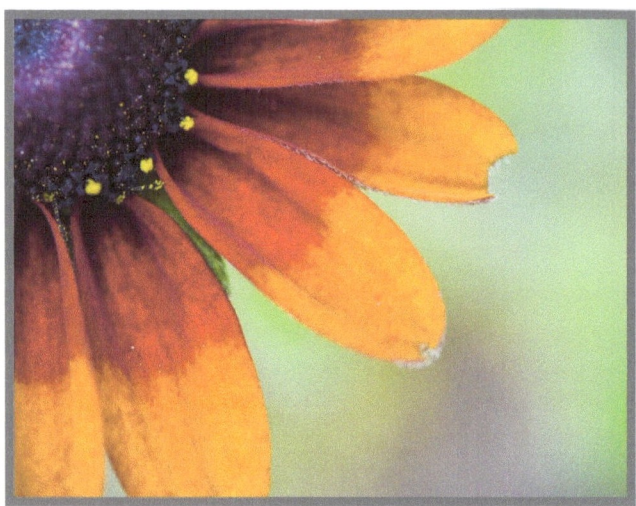

# Acknowledgments

I would like to acknowledge each of my teachers I have had so far in life...

My professors in college and graduate school, my employers, my holistic health and yoga teachers, and most of all, my "life" teachers. Each of you encouraged and inspired me to pursued health, wellness, and disease prevention as a career, and continue to encourage me to pursue learning every day. I especially would like to thank my two amazing kids who bring me joy, love, laughter, health, and beauty every day.

# Table of Contents

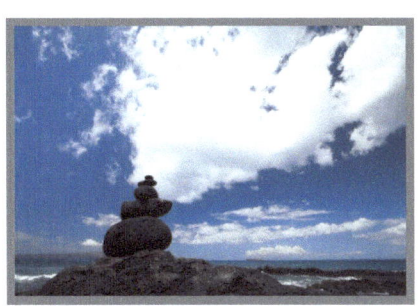

# Welcome to Healthy and Happy Kids

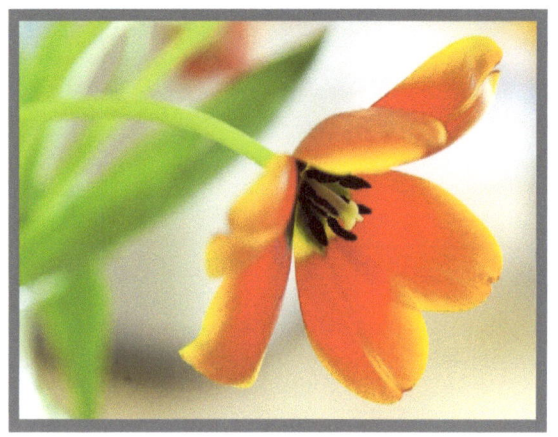

## What is a holistic approach to health?

**Healthy and Happy Kids** is a truly holistic and science-based approach to health that empowers you to teach your kids or students to become healthier by focusing on the health of their body, mind, emotions, and spirit. Many health practices focus mostly on your kids' physical health. While physical health is very important, **Healthy and Happy Kids** also includes tools to help your kids to cope with stress, to believe in themselves, and to feel stronger emotionally. Each of these aspects of health are needed for your kids to be holistically healthy.

## Holistic health for kids

As a parent, you have a lot of roles to play. Raising your kids in health and happiness is extremely important, but isn't always easy. Teaching your kids how to live healthy is time worth spent though, as the healthy habits they develop as kids (eating healthy, moving their body, managing stress) will help them to continue healthy habits as adults. As their bodies grow and mature, their "needs" will change, including hormonal and emotional changes. Similarly, as they experience stress, they may experience health symptoms as a result of their stress. Learning to nourish their body and manage stress and emotions is important for their health.

As healthy aging begins the moment your kids are born, a holistic approach to health is important to include starting at birth, so that your kids can grow healthy and learn skills that can help them to continue to be healthy and happy kids and become healthy and happy adults!

The **Healthy and Happy Kids** workbook is meant to be easy to read and quick to use. This workbook intends to teach and empower **YOU** as a parent, caregiver, or teacher on simple health practices, so that you can then use these skills to help your kids to be as healthy as possible. It does not intend to be a complete book on all health practices available, as that would be a very long and complex book. It also does not aim to be a book on parenting or on discipline. Rather, it focuses on a few of the most important aspects of health for kids.

Now... to truly help your kids to be holistically healthy, you may also want to use this information to enhance your own health, and the health of your entire family. Please feel free to use the information and skills in this wellness workbook to improve aspects of your own health. If you are interested in learning more science-based and holistic health skills than included here, please read *Healthy and Happy for Life!*

# How this workbook is organized

**Healthy and Happy Kids** is written in four sections, including information and exercises on the health of your kid's body, mind, heart, and spirit. Throughout this workbook, each section is briefly discussed, and then a few exercises are suggested to help you and your kids on your way to improved health.

The first time you go through **Healthy and Happy Kids**, you may choose to read the information without doing the exercises. Become familiar with the information. Then go through the workbook again and do the exercises.  You can use the "Notes" page at the end of each section, or a notebook, to take notes.

# Now for a brief disclaimer ...

The information and exercises in the **Healthy and Happy Kids** workbook do not aim to replace the recommendations of your children's physicians, but rather, aim to work along with your medical practitioners. Please have your children continue to have regular visits with their physicians and follow their physicians' instructions. Also make sure their doctors know of any new physical activities or nutritional changes you and your children decide to make.

# Expect success!

Holistic health is not a diet, as diets are temporary. Rather, it is a permanent lifestyle shift. Helping you to empower yourself toward improving your health and your kid's health is the goal of **Healthy and Happy Kids.**

If you have any questions or comments, you can contact me directly at http://BreatheBeWell.com/contact. Enjoy helping your kids to be healthier and happier!

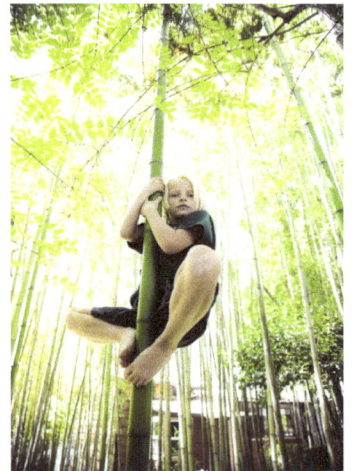

# Section 1: Health of Your Kid's Body

As parents, it is our job to teach our kids early in life to take care of their body, so that they can live the healthiest life possible into old age. This is critically important today as childhood obesity has tripled in the last 30 years and, for the first time in many generations, children born today have a shorter life expectancy than their parents.

This section focuses on skills for your kids to be more physically healthy, including eating healthy food, drinking plenty of water, and moving their bodies. As access to healthy food becomes harder to find, access to unhealthy food has become increasingly easier to find (such as candy at check outs, vending machines, fast food restaurants becoming more common than grocery stores, and drive-thru windows making it possible to get food without doing any physical movement).

Similarly, children today do not have as much access to physical activity, such as physical education in schools and walking or biking to school. At the same time, screen time is becoming increasingly easy to access with computers, tablets, and smart phones available.

With the decreasing access to healthy food and physical activity, and increasing access to unhealthy behaviors, it is important for you as parents to focus on ways to help your children to be more physically healthy.

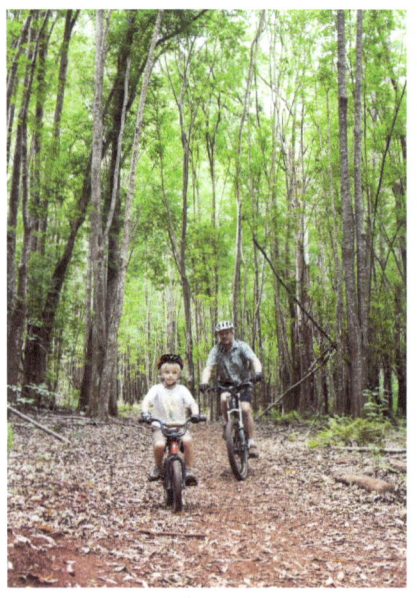

**Please note:** The skills discussed in this workbook should be used in moderation. **Healthy and Happy Kids** does not encourage anyone to aim for perfection, as that isn't realistic and can create stress. As this is a wellness workbook on holistic and balanced health, it is important to LOVE your life as well as live healthy. And yes, this means including foods that you and your kids love every once in a while, even if it is not considered  healthy. There are ways to include unhealthy foods in moderation, in smaller amounts, and as treats rather than as your kid's sole source of food.

# Eat healthy meals and snacks.

Benefits of eating healthy in general include maintaining a healthy weight, increased energy, and preventing many chronic illnesses such as heart disease, stroke, diabetes, and many cancers. For kids specifically, teaching them healthy eating skills will help them to continue to make healthy food decisions as they become adults.

While maintaining a healthy weight and eating a balance of heathy foods are important, I don't believe in diets unless your or your child has food allergies or food sensitivities. This is especially true for children, as they need a healthy balance of all foods, including healthy fats.

**My Plate:** The former Food Pyramid has been replaced with My Plate, which is much easier to understand in terms of planning healthy foods for yourself, your children, and your family.

Basically, My Plate recommends that half of your plate should include a mix of fruits and vegetables. The other half of your plate should include healthy proteins and grains. My Plate also suggests drinking either water or milk with your meals.

Feel free to visit www.ChooseMyPlate.gov/kids for additional information on eating healthy, as well as fun games for kids to play so that they can learn about eating healthy food.

<u>Additional tips to make eating healthy easier</u>

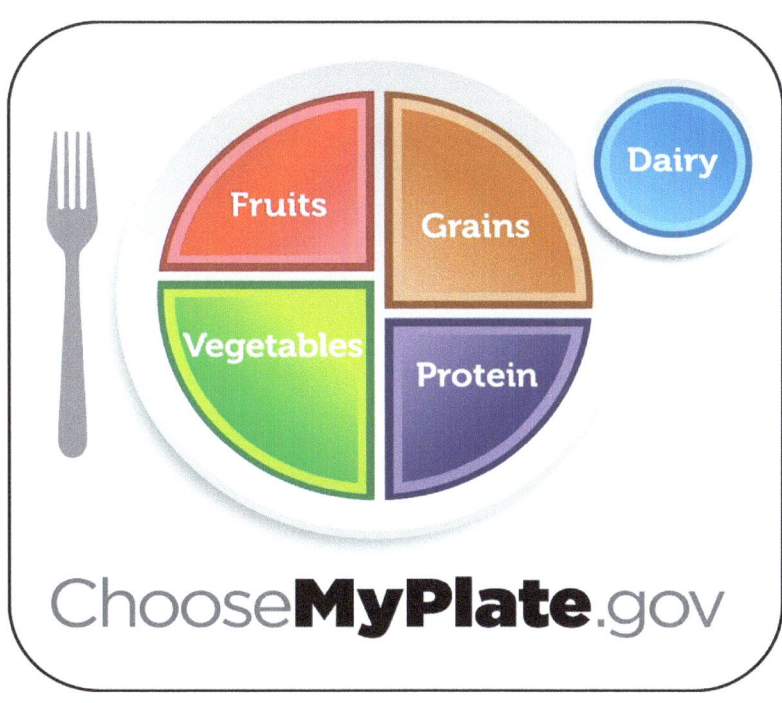

You may be thinking to yourself, "'My Plate' is too simple" or "my kids won't eat vegetables" or "I have no idea where to start." Certain healthy foods not tasting good may be very true for your kids as well as a lot of people. Our bodies and taste buds learn to like the foods we feed ourselves. Luckily though, our bodies and taste buds are able to learn to like new foods. So, if your kids don't like certain healthy foods, choose healthy options that they do like. Over time and as your kids continue to grow, their taste buds may start to like, and even ask for, healthier foods.

Here are a few more suggestions and tips that can make healthy eating easier.

- Include healthy meals and snacks that your kids find tasty and visually appealing. You can get some great recipe ideas at: http://www.choosemyplate.gov/kids/Recipes.html

-  Try to buy foods that are not processed, as processed foods are full of sugar. Sugar is converted to added fat in your kid's body and is one of the leading causes in the obesity epidemic. If sugar is in the first three ingredients in packaged food items, avoid buying them. This may take a bit of effort at first, but effort well spent. You will be amazed at which foods have a lot of added sugar in them.

- Stock your house with healthy and delicious food and snacks. Nuts, fruit, vegetables, yogurt, cheese, baked chips or crackers, and 100% fruit snacks are great snack option.

- Focus on including a variety of fresh fruits, vegetables, healthy grains (such as brown rice, quinoa, and pasta), proteins (such as meat, cheese, beans, legumes, and tofu), and healthy fats (such as olive, flax, hemp, and coconut oil, nuts, fish, and avocado).

- Eat a rainbow of fruits and vegetables. This improves the health effects of food and can make eating healthy more colorful and fun.

- Smoothies, made from fresh fruits and vegetables, are a great way to increase the number of fruits and vegetables your children "eat." You can also add greens, such as kale and spinach, into smoothies and your kids won't even notice.

- Include organic and locally grown food as an additional benefit. Local produce is picked when it is ripe, so it is tastier and has more nutrients when you eat it. Food that is grown locally does not need to be shipped long distances, so it is also better for the environment. Eating locally grown produce also helps to support local farmers, which helps to build your local economy.

- Try to buy foods that are not processed, as processed foods are full of sugar. Sugar is converted to added fat in your kid's body and is one of the leading causes in the childhood obesity epidemic. If sugar is in the first three ingredients in packaged food items, avoid buying them or limit them to special treats. This may take a bit of effort at first, but effort well spent. You will be amazed at which foods have a lot of added sugar in them.

- Foods to keep to a minimum include refined sugar, corn syrup, salt, and saturated fats. ** Be careful to read ingredients on food and beverage packages. There are many products that claim to be "100% fruit," but then list sugar as one of the first three ingredients.

- Include items in meals and snacks that your kids **LOVE**. If these foods are considered to be unhealthy, simply include them as "treats" rather than in their regular meals. Again, you don't need to cut these foods out completely, as it is also important for children to learn to moderate these foods.

- Please do not restrict kid's calories, unless they are actively needing to lose weight, as instructed by their physician. The only calories that should be restricted, are calories from sugar, as these are converted straight into fat. As long as kids are eating well-balanced meals and snacks and moving their bodies, weight should not be an issue.

**\* Exercise**: Make healthy meals and snacks tasty and visually appealing. List at least one healthy meal and one healthy snack that your kids love.

Healthy meal: _____

_____

_____

_____

Healthy snack: _____

_____

_____

**\* Exercise**: Eating healthy is easier when your kids eat what they love. Write down some of your kid's favorite foods, so that you can include them in healthy meals and snacks.

Fruits: _____

_____

_____

Vegetables: _____

_____

Grains: _____

_____

Proteins: _____

_____

**\* Exercise**: Eating a rainbow of fruits and vegetables makes food fun (and colorful). List fruits and vegetables of each color that your kids enjoy eating.

Red: _____

Orange: _____

Yellow: _____

Green: _____

Blue: _____

Purple: _____

**\*Exercise:** Create a three day meal planner.

Use the information from the previous exercises to make a healthy meal and snack plan for three days. Remember to keep it simple and to include a few foods that your kids love as well as healthy foods!

|  | Day One | Day Two | Day Three |
|---|---|---|---|
| **Breakfast** | | | |
| **Snack** | | | |
| **Lunch** | | | |
| **Snack** | | | |
| **Dinner** | | | |
| **Notes:** | | | |

# Drink more water and less sugar-sweetened drinks

Our bodies are roughly 70 percent water, and all parts of our bodies need plenty of it (blood, cells, immune system, brain, organs, and bones). It is recommended to drink at least eight 8-ounce glasses of water every day. This can be challenging for children who aren't used to drinking water or simply don't like the taste of water because they are used to sweeter drink options. Using a water pitcher, with a built-in filtration system built in, and adding flavors, such as lemon or mint, to water can help water to taste better.

It is also highly recommended to limit how many sugar-sweetened beverages your children drink. Sugar-sweetened beverages include soda pop, vitamin water, and sports drinks, to name a few. Sugar is converted into fat in your kid's body and has no nutritional value. Simply put, we can drink much more sugar than we can eat and. As each 12 ounce soda includes 16 tablespoons of sugar, drinking just one sugar drink per day can add eight pounds of weight per year in youth and 15 pounds of weight per year in adults. Hence, sugar drinks are among the culprits leading to the rising obesity and diabetes rates in children.

If your children enjoy sugar-sweetened drinks, try to only include these beverages in moderation, as excess sugar is not good for their health. One suggestion is to limit sugar drinks to special occasions, rather than drinking them on a regular basis.

**\* Exercise:** Tools for drinking more water and less sugar-sweetened beverages.

What are your kid's drink preferences?

_____

List challenges for your kids to drink eight glasses of water each day.

_____

List challenges to cutting back on sugar drinks.

_____

List at least one way you can increase access to water.

_____

List at least one way you can cut back on sugar drinks.

_____

# Kids need to move their bodies at least 60 minutes <u>every</u> day

Access to physical activity is becoming harder to find, especially with decreases in physical education in the schools and fewer children walking or riding their bikes to school. At the same time, access to "screen time" is becoming easier to get. Children need to move their bodies a minimum of 60 minutes every day. However, national data suggests that many children are not meeting this recommendation.

Physical activity helps your kids to maintain a healthy weight, helps their immune systems to stay healthy, helps to prevent many chronic diseases and forms of cancer, helps them to focus and concentrate in school, and helps improve their emotional health and self-confidence.

All forms of physical activity are good for your children (and for you). Physical activity does not need to be an organized activity. It can be as simple as jumping on a trampoline, kicking a ball with a friend or parent, a game of tag, playing at the beach, exploring in the park, or walking a dog.

Make physical activity something your kids love! Swimming, biking, running, playing soccer, or simply playing with friends are just a few examples. If your children do what they love, they will be more likely to continue to be physically active their entire lives.

Do something active together as a family that is fun for everyone. This way you can all have fun together and you can get some exercise too!

Finally, minimize screen time. Our bodies burns fewer calories watching TV than while doing <u>absolutely nothing</u>. Limit TV and screen time to a set maximum amount each day (preferably less than one hour). Or save screen time for bad weather days or special occasions.

**\* Exercise:** What are some of your kids favorite physical activities to do and what are some activities your family can enjoy doing together?

Your kids' favorite activities: _____

_____

_____

_____

_____

_____

_____

Days and times your kids can do activities : _____

Physical activities the whole family can enjoy doing together: _____

_____

_____

_____

_____

_____

_____

Days and times you and your kids can do activities together: _____

# Oral health

Oral health is important as the mouth is the first step in the digestive process and digestive health. And digestive health is an important part of the immune system and your kid's ability to fight germs. So, good oral health can help your kids to fight off infections and to live healthier.

It is important for kids to start seeing a dentist and have regular dental cleanings and exams once they have teeth. Proper daily oral hygiene includes brushing (especially after meals) and flossing, which helps to clear bacteria trapped between the teeth and gums. There are wonderful devices on the market, such as electric toothbrushes and flossing aids that help make brushing and flossing for children easier and more fun.

If your children have challenges or health concerns related to their oral health (such as cavities, gum disease, or gum swelling, bleeding, or discomfort), it is important to follow up with their dentist. Resolving these issues will help improve their immune system and overall health.

**\*Exercise:** Tools for improving dental health.

Which aspect of dental health would you like to help your kids to improve?

(for example: more brushing, daily flossing, seeing the dentist more regularly)

_____

_____

List challenges to improving your kid's dental health.

_____

_____

List one step you can take to help improve your kid's dental health.

(for example: get a new toothbrush or flossing aids)

_____

_____

# Get plenty of sleep and "down" time

Kids can have very busy schedules between school, homework, sports, after school activities, play dates, household chores, and family time. It is important that they get plenty of sleep and down time, so they can rest and reconnect with themselves. Once kids stop taking naps, reading a book is a great way to get down time or quiet time. At first, if you kids aren't used to having down time, they may get a bit bored. This is OK. Boredom is actually good for kids. Often times, being bored leads to increased imagination. It's amazing what kids can come up with when they get bored and their imagination kicks in.

\* This topic is also discussed in Section 4, **Health of your Kid's Spirit** on page 32.

**\*Exercise:** Opportunities for "down time"

List times of the day where your children can get some "down time."

_____

_____


# Reward system

Set up a reward system where your children can earn marbles (or some other token) for good behaviors, and include a chart of items (rewards) that your children can "buy" after earning these tokens. These reward items can be small (for short-term goals) or large (for larger steps taken or reaching their final goal).

Simply place a marble in the jar each time your children earns one by doing one of the below behaviors.

Behaviors to earn marbles

List behaviors for each marble earned (for example: eating vegetables, drinking water, using kind words, or doing their chores).

1 marble earned:

_____

_____

_____

_____

## Rewards to spend their marbles on and what these rewards cost

List rewards and how many marbles they costs.

Cost 1 marble:

_____

_____

_____

_____

Cost 5 marbles:

_____

_____

_____

_____

Cost 10 marbles:

_____

_____

_____

_____

Rewards for when your children reach a larger or final goal:

_____

_____

_____

_____

_____

# Notes page

Write down notes about what you learned in this section, and how it relates to you, your kids, and your family.

# Section 2: Health of Your Kid's Mind

The mind is an amazing entity that can assist your kids in moving forward toward their goals, can help them to cope with stress, and can affect how they perceive the world as either positive or negative.

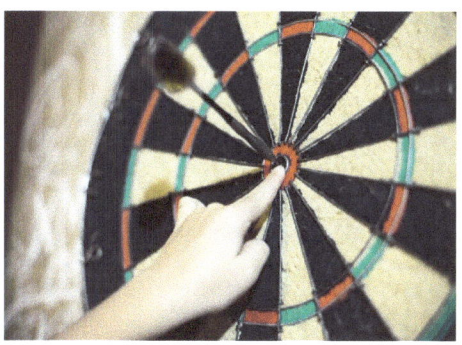

Stress, anxiety, and depression can have a large and profoundly negative effect on your kids' health. Hence, it's important to make the health of your kids' mind (stress reduction) one of your top priorities.

This section provides a few simple skills to help your kids (and you) to cope with, and minimize, the effects of stress in their lives. This way, your kids can better view life as positive, be less fearful of potentially stressful events, and become the best that they can be.

## What is stress and how can it affect your kids?

Stress can be <u>any change</u> in life. It can be positive change as well as negative change. Stress can even be imagined or anticipated change. Stress can affect your kid's physical health, and their thoughts and emotions. Stress can also create anxiety and depression and affect the quality of your kid's school work, their friendships, self-confidence, and their enjoyment in life. Given that change is the one constant in life, unfortunately then, so is stress. By helping your kids to cope with stress, they will be better able to deal with life's changes in a healthy way.

Here are a few examples of situations that can create stress in your kid's life:

- Illness or death in the family

- School challenges or issues being bullied

- Moving or having friends move away

- Divorce

- A new baby

- Simply growing up (physical changes, hormone changes, emotional changes)

- Exams in school or competitions in extra-curricular activities

# A – B – C's (Affirmations, Belly breathing, and Coping skills)

As parents, it is our job to teach our kids new skills, while at the same time, to love them for who they are and boost their self-confidence. This can be tough to accomplish, but is important for developing healthy kids.

The A – B – C's (Affirmations, Belly breathing, and Coping skills) are simply a few tools for you, as a parent, to keep in your "tool kit" to help with creating positive behaviors and creating healthy and positive kids.

## "A" - Affirmations

Your kid's thoughts, or self-talk, create their words. Their words create their actions, which then lead to their habits. By helping your kids to create positive thoughts, you are helping them to believe in themselves, learn new skills, and create positive events in their present life and in their future.  Affirmations, or positive self-talk, help kids learn new behaviors or change old habits, while at the same time, boosting their self-esteem. When you help your kids to write or say affirmations, it is important to keep the affirmations positive and in the present-tense (such as "I am…" or "I am willing to…" rather than "I want to be…" or "I don't want to be…" ).

How do these words make you feel? How do they make your kids feel?

I'm stupid        I'm weak        I'm no good        I have no friends

I'm ugly        My life sucks

Write down how these words may make your kids feel:

_____

Now... How do these words make you feel? How do they make your kids feel?

I am smart        I am brave        I am strong        I am loved!

I'm beautiful        I can do anything        I am enough

Write down how these words may make your kids feel:

_____

**\* Exercise:** Help your kids to create positive affirmations.

Start by teaching your children self-loving statements: "I love myself" and "I am the perfect 'me' just as I am."

Next, ask your kids to complete the statement "I am... " with all of the positive qualities that they are. And you can definitely help them out by letting them know all of the wonderful qualities you feel they are.

"I am... "

_____

_____

_____

_____

_____

Now set one positive affirmation to help improve a behavior each of your kids are ready to work on:

"I am ready and able to... (fill in the blank with skills your child is ready to do) ...

For example: "I am ready and able to focus on my homework and finish it without distraction."

_____

_____

_____

_____

_____

Here is one of my favorite affirmations for kids and adults...

*"I am braver than I believe, stronger than I seem, and smarter than I think"*

~ Christopher Robin to Winnie the Pooh

In addition to learning to talk to themselves positively, it's important for your kids to hear positive statements from you. Let your kids know that you believe in them and that they can do anything they put their mind to. You are your kid's hero. You believing in their success is very important!

**\* Exercise:**  How you talk to your kids.

Here are some suggestions of statements your kids need to hear from you, so that they can learn to talk to themselves more positively and can learn to believe in themselves.

- *I love you*
- *I am grateful for you*
- *When you do _____, you make me happy*
- *I am proud of you*
- **I believe in you!**

Also, it's important to be aware of how you talk to your kids when they have done something wrong. Here are a few steps to follow so that you and your kids can have positive conversations and have a positive outcome.

- Be specific about what they have done wrong <u>right now</u>. Avoid bringing up things they have done wrong in the past.
- Together, set a goal that can improve the issue from happening again. Help them learn from their mistakes.
- Ask your child for his or her ideas on how to work toward reaching this goal.
- Set a goal date and time (if applicable) and then follow up with your child on their progress.
- Set a reward for achieving this positive goal.

Let your kids know that all kids, and people of all ages, have challenges and lessons to learn. Other people's challenges may be different than the challenges in front of your kids, but everyone has them. This step is important as it lets your kids know that they are not alone, or different from others, simply because they have challenges or things to improve. Finally, tell your kids that you love them and that you believe in them regardless of when they do something wrong.

# "B" - Belly breathing

Breathing is not only the source of life, but it also helps your kids to stay calm during stressful situations. The breath also fuels their brain, so they can think more effectively (which is great for school and tests) and can cope better during stressful situations. And of course, the breath can be used to help prevent a situation from becoming stressful. Especially when combined with positive self-talk. The best part of the breath is it's **FREE** and always available to you and your kids!

**\* Exercise:** Belly breathing.

Practice this exercise so you can then teach it to your kids.

- Sit comfortably and place one hand on your belly and the other hand on your chest.
- Close your eyes and breathe with your mouth closed.
- Now, imagine there is a balloon in your belly. Fill up the balloon with your breath. After you have inhaled completely, slowly exhale the air out of the balloon.
- After several breaths, you can focus on lengthening the length of your breaths, especially your exhales, so that you are breathing slower.

You can teach this simple breathing skill to your children. First have your children take a few belly breaths. Then ask them to make each breath longer.

If your children have worries, they can add this step:

- Have them close their eyes and visualize their worries going into the balloon as they breathe in. Once the balloon is filled up with their worries, they can release the balloon (along with their worries) when they are done and feel relaxed.

That's it! Simple.

## "C" - Coping skills

Coping skills use the breathing skills you just practiced, combined with positive self-talk, to help your kids to get through stressful situations with ease.

Practice these steps so that you can teach them to your kids. Then they can use them any time they notice their body, mind, or emotions feeling stressed.

1. Say to yourself, either out loud or in your mind, "**STOP!**" (to negative thoughts, beliefs, feelings, frustrations, or worries you may be having). Saying **"STOP"** to yourself acts as a jolt to break yourself out of this potential downward spiral of negative thinking.

2. **Breathe deep into your belly** as you just learned (and again... and again...) until your heart rate slows, your inhalations and exhalations slow and balance out, your muscles relax, and your negative thoughts or worries slow down.

3. **Pat yourself on the back** for how far you've come, and simply for noticing and working on reducing stress. It isn't always easy to recognize that you are experiencing stress, let alone work on it. It is even harder for your kids. So please applaud their efforts as they learn these skills too.

4. Depending on what the stressful situation is, **think of just one next step** you can do to move toward a solution. You do not need to come up with an entire solution. Just one step! And if you can't think of a next step, your next step can always be to ask someone else for help. You can teach your kids that, if they need, their next step can be asking you, their teacher, or another adult for help.

5. Finally, go do something fun! Yes, simply stop what you were doing, even for just five minutes, and do something fun. This lightens the mood. When you are ready, you can go back to what you were doing with a new outlook. :)

**\* Exercise:** Now it's time to practice.

Close your eyes and visualize a stressful situation. Use the above steps to calm yourself, so that you can experience the positive effects before teaching this exercise to your kids.

# Additional tools for teaching kids positive outlook on life

## Help your children to perceive the world as positive

With your kids, start off the day with a big hug! Next, talk with them about how today is going to be a great day. Take a moment to notice everything positive in that moment. Ask your kids what they notice around them that is positive and what they are looking forward today.

**\* Exercise:** Living in the moment.

Again, practice this exercise so you can then teach it to your kids...

- Notice all there is around you: what are you seeing, hearing, smelling, tasting, feeling in your body, and feeling emotionally.

- What is joyful about these things you are noticing?

- What are you looking forward to today?

This exercise can help set the stage for your children to have a great day!

## Create a positive and calm environment for your kids, your family, and yourself

By creating pleasant, positive, and calm environments, it is easier to view the world as positive. Here are a few simple suggestions for creating positive environments for you and your kids:

- De-clutter your home. By simplifying your space, it becomes more relaxing and less stressful. It is also then easier to keep clean, which is healthier for everyone.

- Play pleasant and fun music.

- Buy or pick flowers to place in your home.

- Do some arts and crafts together.

- Create plenty of opportunities for giggle time. Laughter is the best medicine for calming the mind!

- Create signs or notes for your kids that include positive affirmations and messages. Hang the signs in their rooms and place notes in their lunch boxes.

## A few more skills for a healthy mind...

Catch your kids being good! It isn't always easy, but it is important for their health and for your relationship with your kids.

Avoid saying "NO." What did I just suggest? I am not suggesting that you say "yes" to everything your kids want. But the word "NO" is final. It doesn't offer an alternative or a middle area where there are options. Here are some options instead of saying a flat out "no."

- Offer a later time: If you are busy and your kids want your attention, ask them to wait 10 minutes (or another amount of time). This way you are still saying "yes" and letting them know that they are important to you.

- Offer an alternative: If they are asking for something unhealthy (such as candy), you can offer them an alternative option that is still tasty but healthier. So, again, you are still saying "yes."

- Let your kids come up with a solution... For example, if they are asking to buy something that is expensive, ask your kid to come up with some ideas on how he or she can make the money.

Give your kids the gift of time and fun with you, which is much more valuable than "things." Invest in your kids by being approachable and listening to them when they want or need to talk.

Follow through on your promises!

Give your kids what they NEED, not what they deserve. This isn't always easy, but kids are just that... kids. They are still learning and figuring out life. They make mistakes and need help. So, even if you feel they don't deserve help, give them help because they need help.

Along the line of giving your kids what they need, also give your kids a second chance. Or even a third, fourth, and fifth chance... We all make mistakes and are imperfect. Kids, especially, need to know that you believe in them by giving them another chance.

*"You are braver than you believe, stronger than you seem,*

*and smarter than you think"*

# Notes page

Write down notes about what you learned in this section, and how it relates to you, your kids, and your family.

# Section 3: Health of Your Kid's Heart

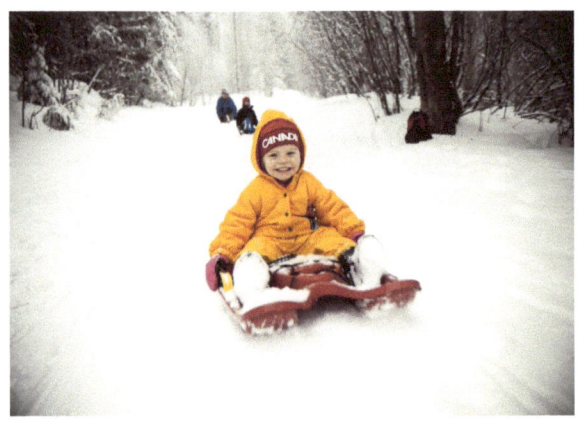

We can only extend love to others if we first love ourselves.

How you love your kids, will profoundly affect how their tender hearts grows, will affect their self-esteem, and will affect how they then love and treat others. Helping to build self-love in your kids will then help them to believe that they are deserving of healthy and happy relationships and will help them to stay away from unhealthy relationships.

## Love your kids for who they are!

Love your kids for who they are, right now. Write down each of your kid's positive qualities and remind them of these qualities often. It is easy to focus on what we want our children to learn. Remember to first, and more importantly, celebrate who they are today!

**\* Exercise**: List positive qualities of each of your kids.

This is an important exercise, so we're going to do it again. List positive qualities of each of your kids.

_____

_____

_____

_____

**\* Exercise:** Have your children list positive qualities about themselves.

Now, ask each of your kids to list positive qualities about themselves.

_____

_____

_____

_____

# Nightly gratitudes

Kids are never too young to learn how many things they have in their lives to be grateful for, including their family, friends, home, siblings, pets, school, health, food, love, laughter, toys... the list goes on.

Being grateful has many benefits:

- Improves their outlook on life and your level of happiness.
- Reduces stress, anxiety, and depression.
- Actually creates positive experiences and more things to be grateful for!

To help your kids to focus on what they are grateful for, end each day by asking them:

- What they love about themselves (and tell them what **YOU** love about them as well).
- To list the things for which they are grateful.

# Positive messages and love notes

Surround your kids with positive messages. Here are a few suggestions.

- Write positive messages on a white board or chalk board.
- Write positive messages on extra paper or grocery bags. Hang them in their rooms.
- Place love notes in their lunch boxes. At any age, kids love to be loved and acknowledged.

# Do something they love

Include time for something your kids love, just because... Do something together. Let your kids choose the activity. Remember, time spent with your kids is way more important than spending money on them.

**\* Exercise:** List a few ideas of things you can do with your kids.

_____

_____

# Follow their dreams and believe in themselves

Always encourage your kids to follow their dreams, no matter how silly they may seem to you. By learning and believing they can do <u>anything</u>, they will always know that the sky is the limit.

# Volunteer or simply do something kind for others

At any age, encourage your kids to volunteer. Depending on the ages of your kids, volunteering can be done at an organization or simply by helping around the house, helping a neighbor, or taking care of a pet (even if just a gold fish). Helping others helps your kids to feel better about themselves AND has been shown to improve their health.

**\* Exercise:** List a couple of ways your kids can volunteer or help someone else.

_____

_____

# Allow your kids to feel ALL emotions

We have learned to label being happy as "good" and being afraid, sad, or angry as "bad." Emotions are simply emotions and they each have their place in life. It is healthier for your kids to allow themselves to feel all emotions and learn healthy ways to cope with them. When your kids are sad, let them cry. When they are afraid, let them talk about their fears. When angry, they can hit a pillow, scream into a pillow, or go run. Once they are calm, they can talk about what made them angry. It is much healthier, in the long run, to express all emotions, in a healthy way. Then they can let them go, rather than bottle them up just for the emotions to come out stronger in the future.

All of this said, it is sometimes hard and stressful for us parents to watch our children be sad, afraid, or angry. This may be a good time for you to also learn healthy ways to cope with and manage your emotions and stress. Feel free to use some of the skills in this workbook to improve your own health, if you wish.

Additionally, if you have a child who often times gets very emotional, it is okay to suggest that they let out their emotions alone for a few minutes. This may help you to better cope with your emotions as well. Once your child has expressed himself fully, you can help him or her use their breath and coping skills learned in the previous section.

Finally, it's good to end these emotional moments by lightening up the mood by doing something fun and relaxing together.

# Notes page

Write down notes about what you learned in this section, and how it relates to you, your kids, and your family.


*** Unfortunately, many adults have challenges with self-love.*

*Teaching kids early to love themselves is important,*

*so they can grow into loving adults! ***

# Section 4: Health of Your Kid's Spirit

If all children learned to meditate at a young age, the world would be a much more peaceful place...

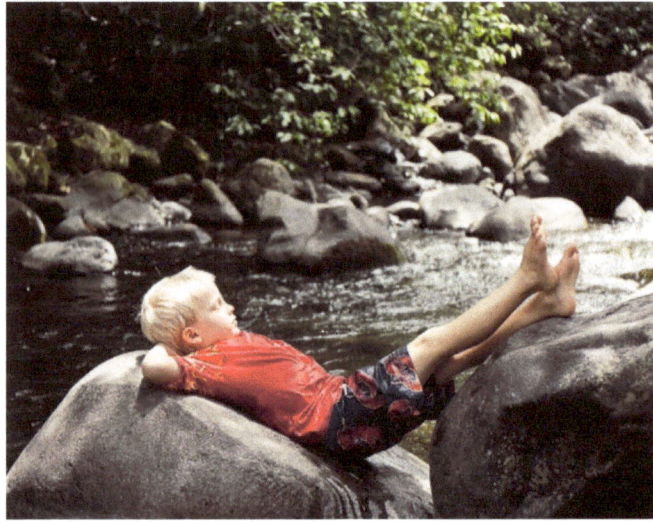

## Benefits of meditation

Spending time being quiet can help your children to:

- have a clear and uncluttered mind
- stay calm
- become centered and in the present moment
- have less agitation, anxiety, and stress
- be less reactive
- think of solutions with ease
- have more energy
- have a healthier immune system
- reconnect to themselves

By spending time being completely quiet, your children can learn to have a calm awareness and "intuition" as to whether a situation is healthy and positive or unhealthy and potentially dangerous. With this calm awareness, your kids can then choose to walk away from negative situations, such as in the event of peer pressure.

If meditation is new to your child, have him start off by meditating for just a few minutes each day and build up slowly over time. Encourage your child to be kind to himself during meditation. Make it a "judgement-free" zone. It is normal for thoughts to enter our mind. Teach your child to simply acknowledge these thoughts and then release them with his breath, without grabbing on to them and without judgment. Just like a river, notice them and then let them pass. There are many types of meditation practices, depending on your child's personality and preferences. But any form of meditation, which allows his mind to be quiet, calm, and free of rules, will help him to reap the benefits of meditation. After a period of time of regular meditation practice, your child may be surprised at how calm and clear his mind becomes. Below are a few suggestions for different types of meditation practices. Try doing meditation together as a family!

# Spend time in quiet

Quiet time does not mean TV or computer games, as these activities do not allow your kid's mind to quiet down. Here are a few suggestions on how your kids can positively create quiet time:

Sitting meditation. Have your kids sit comfortably, either in a chair or on pillows on the floor. Have them close their eyes and simply breathe and be still for a few minutes at a time. If this is a new practice for them, they can start with two minutes and slowly build up to 15 minutes or longer.

Laying meditation (called Savasana in yoga) is another option for quiet time. Have your kids lay on their back on the floor with their arms and legs comfortably stretched out. If they like, they can cover their eyes with a cloth or eye pillow to make the room dark. Just be careful they don't fall asleep.

Walking or swimming meditation. Your kids can also spend time in quiet while walking or swimming. Walking meditation is best done in quiet, without listening to music, texting, or communicating with others in any other way. It is also ideally done in a pleasant environment away from traffic and noise, if possible. Your kids can also choose to do swimming meditation at a pool. It is calming to just focus on the black line at the bottom of the pool.

Yoga. Yoga is another form of moving meditation. Yoga is also a good activity to help calm kids when they get over-excited, to build self-confidence, and to stay centered before taking tests. There are several kids yoga decks, DVD's, and YouTube videos available on-line, so that kids can practice yoga at home. Simply search on-line for "yoga for kids" or "kid's yoga decks." Many yoga studios also include classes for kids. You can check with your local yoga studios for yoga classes for kids.

Creative meditation. Art and dance can be forms of creative meditation, including drawing, painting, free-form dance, music, or acting, just to name a few... The key creative meditation is to simply let the art come out of you naturally, without rules and restrictions.

Mantra to clear your mind. Regardless of which form of quiet time or meditation your children choose, they can add a mantra to help clear their mind. Mantras can be any word or phrase that has personal meaning to them. If they do not have a personal mantra, they can start by using the word "ohm." As any thoughts come in, simply let them pass through without judgment.

# Spend time in nature

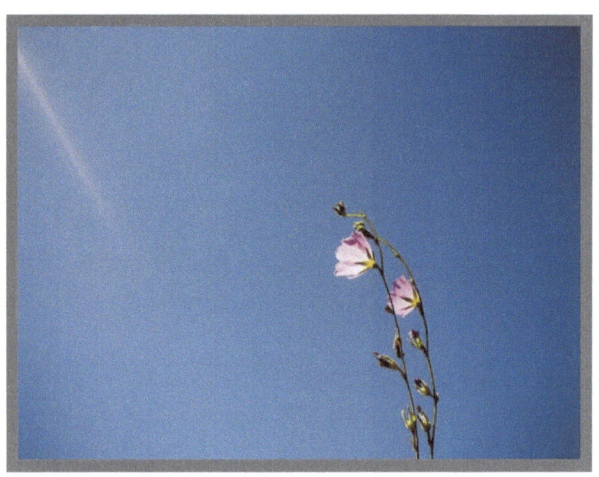

Spending time in nature can help your kids to connect to the source of life, so they can become both energized and calm and centered at the same time. Depending on where you live, here are a few suggestions on places where you and your kids can connect with nature:

- Beach

- Forest

- Desert

- Oceans, lakes and rivers

- Parks and gardens

- Mountains

- Open fields

- Snow

- Anywhere there is nature (fresh air, trees, grass, flowers and plants, dirt, water or animals) and where your kids can hear and smell the natural sounds and smells of the earth.

**\* Exercise**: List at least one place you plan to spend time in nature with your kids this week.

_____

_____

# Additional tools helpful for improving the health of the spirit

Depending on your family's beliefs, you and your kids can also spend time in religious or spiritual practice. Examples include spending time in prayer, stating blessings for things your children are grateful for in their lives, or simply sending out well wishes to others.

"Spending time in quiet and simply 'being' is important so that you can receive messages from the universe and from your own body"

# Notes page

Write down notes about what you learned in this section, and how it relates to you, your kids, and your family.

# Bonus Tips for Raising Healthy and Happy Kids

### It's OK to make mistakes

Teach your kids that it's okay to make mistakes. The important thing is to simply try!

### See the humor in situations

Teach your kids the art of laughing at themselves and seeing humor in situations. Show them by example the next time you make a mistake at something or accidentally do something silly. Or share a story about a time when you made a mistake and how finding humor in it helped you to laugh rather than feel embarrassed.

### Expect regression

Expect  set-backs in your kids and in yourself! None of us are perfect. And especially with important behavior changes, set-backs are part of the process.

### Other tips?

What other tips can you think of that would help your children and your family to become healthier?

_____

_____

_____

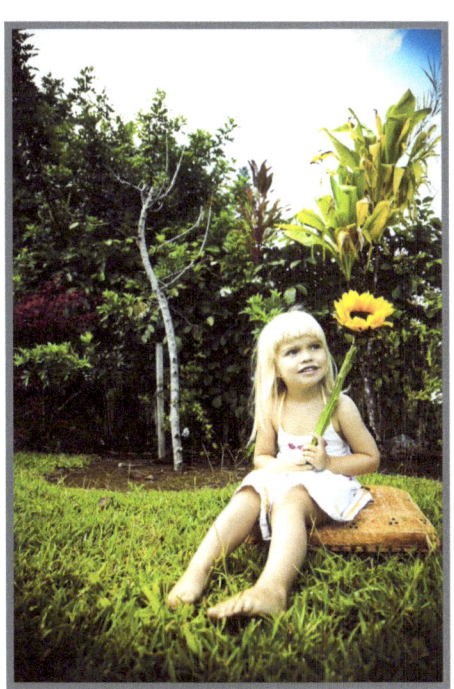

# Notes page

Write down notes about what you learned in this section, and how it relates to you, your kids, and your family.

activity in the Arctic region remains dangerous, a decrease in both ice coverage and ice

thickness does allow for increased access to areas not accessible in the past.[5] These factors

have led to the opening of maritime shipping routes which can potentially decrease transit

times across the globe.

## Arctic Circumnavigation Route Map

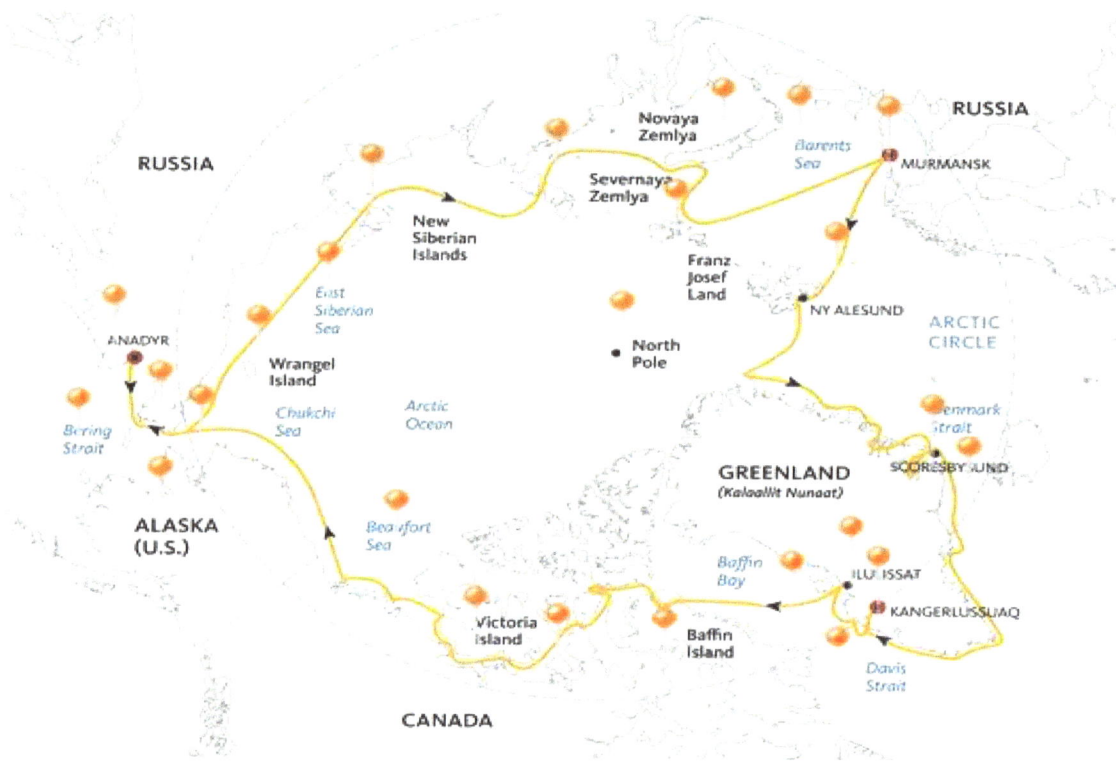

Figure 1.[6]

In addition to shipping, the retreat of sea ice in the Arctic has led to an increase in

fishing vessels venturing farther north and staying longer in those waters. Between 2008 and

2010, fishing in the Arctic increased by 44%, with most of that occurring in the Barents and

---

4 "An estimated 34% decrease in annual mean ice thickness since 1980." Michael D. Bowes, *Impact of Climate Change on Naval Operations in the Arctic*, (CNA: 2009), 6, document can be obtained through the Defense Technical Information Center at www.dtic.mil.

5 In 2008, for the first time in recorded history, the Northwest Passage, winding through the Canadian Archipelago, and the Northern Sea Route, running along the northern coast of Russia, were available for open water transit. Ibid, p 4.

6 Craig Lloyd, "Coast Guard District 17 Arctic Brief" (Brief presented at the Naval War College Fleet Arctic Operations Game, Newport, RI, September 13, 2011).

# About the Author

Congratulations on taking your first step toward learning tips for helping your kids to live healthier, holistically. You are on your way to a helping your kids, yourself, and your family to live a lifetime of health and happiness! I'm excited for you!

I have been working in health and wellness for over 25 years. I have two masters degrees in health-related fields. One in Cardiovascular Epidemiology (The study of heart health, obesity prevention, and healthy aging) from Stanford University, and another in Behavioral Psychology from University of the Pacific. I also spent several years working in healthy aging and quality-of-life at U.C. San Francisco, Institute for Healthy Aging.

During my many years working in health, wellness, and health research, I have worn many hat. Including health and weight loss counseling, chronic disease self-management, using breath, visualization, and biofeedback to manage stress, studying what motivates people to take part in healthy behaviors, healthy aging, quality-of-life, spirituality and health, and helping high-risk groups to learn healthy behaviors. Upon moving to Hawaii, I changed my focus briefly to helping to create healthier communities. I have worked with many types of people to live healthier lives. I love everything to do with helping people to live healthier and happier.  **I LOVE what I do!**

I am the founder and owner of *Breathe & Be Wellness* and developed **Healthy and Happy for Life!** And **Happy and Healthy Kids,** which is based on my many years working in health and wellness, and learning what really worked for people to become healthier. This includes foremost, empowering people to help themselves with skills and knowledge, removing rules about how to be healthy, and including a holistic approach to health.

**I am a mom of two beautiful kids, who give my life a whole new meaning.** I use the tools and exercises in this workbook to help myself and my kids to be the healthiest and happiest we can possibly be.

My passion in life is to help all people to become healthier. I feel that health can be very simple and easy to attain when a holistic approach is used.

I hope **Healthy and Happy for Kids** is helpful for you and your family's health. If you are interested in improving your own health, I invite you to read **Healthy and Happy for Life!**

If you have any questions or comments, please feel free to contact me directly at http://breathebewell.com/contact/.

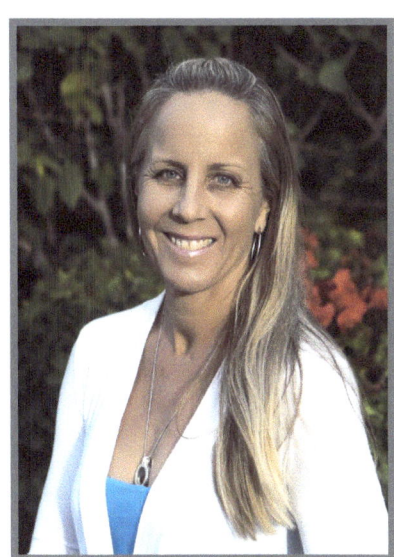

In health and happiness,   **Kristin M Mills, MS, MA**
*Breathe & Be Wellness*

www.ingramcontent.com/pod-product-compliance
Lightning Source LLC
Chambersburg PA
CBHW060839290526
45792CB00006BB/1987